APPLE CIDER
VINEGAR

The Complete Guide to
sApple Cider Vinegar

SUSAN GREY

Grow Your Pantry Are On A Mission

To get 2,000,000 people to grow their own food over the next 10 years...

How will we help 2,000,000 people reconnect to their food?

Free online resources, affordable kitchen products, affordable growing products

For free ebooks on growing your own food, recipes and how to guides just visit our website and enter your email at:

www.growyourpantry.com

Once you've signed up to our exclusive emailing list you will receive your first free e-book!

Between our online resource centre and free content delivered to you weekly via email be sure to not miss out...

Table of Contents

Introduction

Due to a variety of factors, such as hectic schedules, lack of money, and limited knowledge regarding healthy living, people tend to consume unhealthy food products.

Instead of preparing and cooking their own meals at home, they turn to processed goods, junk food, fast food, and fatty foods because they are less expensive and easier to access.

It's understandable that people work hard to make enough money to sustain their necessities. However, this is not a good reason to neglect health and wellness. See to it that you eat nutritious foods such as fruits, vegetables, lean meats, and whole wheats. Avoid microwavable foods, canned and bottled foods, take outs, and other unhealthy food choices.

If you do not want to suffer from chronic illnesses such as cancers, diabetes, and high blood pressure, you should consider using apple cider vinegar.

Hippocrates, the father of medicine, was the first to promote the benefits of apple cider vinegar. Today, numerous studies support claims regarding the benefits and effectiveness of this fascinating tonic. It has even been scientifically proven to be effective in helping treat medical conditions as well as improve them.

But vinegar does not taste good! Why should I include it in my regular diet?

You may have doubts and concerns about using apple cider vinegar, especially if you do not like its taste.

Well, there's no need to be alarmed. If you are concerned about not having a pleasant experience due to its strong acidic taste, you can always include it as an ingredient to your meals or beverages rather than drinking it straight.

And yes, you will find a list of recipes that you can use in this book. See to it that you follow these recipes to enjoy and benefit from them. Rest assured that you'll find apple cider vinegar to be an amazing ingredient. And it isn't hard to find. You can find apple cider vinegar online, in supermarkets, and in health food stores.

Start changing your life today. Begin by learning about this special kind of vinegar and using it to detoxify, energize, and improve your body.

Apple cider vinegar is generally safe to use, provided that the dosage does not go above two tablespoons per day. If you have certain health conditions, make sure that you consult your doctor before taking it in any form.

CHAPTER 1:
The Basics of Apple Cider Vinegar

Apple cider vinegar, also known as cider vinegar, is a fermented juice that comes from crushed apples. It contains vitamins B1, B2, B6, and C as well as pectin, folic acid, biotin, pantothenic acid, and niacin. It also has minerals such as sodium, iron, magnesium, calcium, phosphorus, and potassium. Plus, it's loaded with citric acid and acetic acid.

Why Apple Cider Vinegar?

The so-called natural tonic has high acetic acid content and potent biological effects. Its production involves a two-step process. First, apples are crushed and exposed to yeast. This ferments their sugars and converts them into alcohol. Then, bacteria are added to this alcohol solution to ferment it further and convert it into acetic acid, which is the primary active compound of vinegars.

Organic, unfiltered apple cider vinegar contains mother, which are strands of enzymes, proteins, and good bacteria that make the product appear murky. According to some, the benefits of apple cider vinegar mostly come from the mother. There are plenty of reasons why you should use this product:

Apple cider vinegar can kill different types of harmful bacteria.

It contains acetic acid, which can prevent bacteria from multiplying. You can use it to clean and disinfect your home, as well as treat ear infections, warts, nail fungus, and lice. It can also be used to preserve food naturally.

Apple cider vinegar can fight against diabetes and lower blood sugar levels.

You can use it to manage diabetes. Type-2 diabetes is generally characterized by high levels of blood sugar caused by an inability to produce insulin or insulin resistance.

Apple cider vinegar can improve insulin sensitivity by nineteen to thirty-four percent as well as reduce blood sugar by thirty-four percent after consuming fifty grams of white bread. Moreover, it can reduce blood sugar by four percent.

It is ideal to use apple cider vinegar if you are pre-diabetic, diabetic, or simply want to maintain low blood sugar levels. Again, however, if you are using certain medications for your condition, see to it that you consult your doctor beforehand.

Apple cider vinegar can help you reduce belly fat and lose weight.

According to studies, vinegar contains properties that aid in weight loss. It can increase your satiety so that you will consume fewer calories. For instance, you may take apple cider vinegar with a high-carb meal to feel full faster. This allows you to reduce your calorie intake by 200 to 275.

In a study that involved 175 obese individuals, it was found that consuming apple cider vinegar can lead to weight loss and reduced belly fat. Those who consumed one tablespoon of the product lost 1.2 kilograms, while those who consumed two tablespoons lost 1.7 kilograms.

Apple cider vinegar can improve heart health and lower cholesterol.

Statistics have shown that heart disease is the leading cause of premature death in the world. When you consume apple cider vinegar, you reduce the risk factors associated with heart disease.

Apple cider vinegar has been found to lower triglyceride and cholesterol levels, as well as reduce blood pressure, which is a common cause of kidney problems and heart diseases. Moreover, apple cider vinegar can help fight against diabetes, lower blood sugar levels, and improve insulin sensitivity, which are all risk factors for heart disease.

Apple cider vinegar can help fight against cancers.

Cancer is typically characterized by uncontrolled cell growth. According to studies, apple cider vinegar contains anti-cancer properties. It can help shrink tumors and kill cancer cells. In fact, its intake has been linked to decreased esophageal cancer.

On the Matter of Use and Dosage

Apple cider vinegar is most ideal for cooking and preparing food. It is best for homemade mayonnaise, salad dressings, and meals. It can also be diluted in water and consumed as a beverage. As much as possible, you should opt for organic, unfiltered apple cider vinegar that contains the mother.

The usual dosages of apple cider vinegar range from one to two teaspoons to one to two tablespoons per day. It should be mixed in a glass of water. It must also be taken in small doses at first. Refrain from taking large amounts of apple cider vinegar. Too much of this product can result in unpleasant and possibly dangerous side effects.

The appropriate dosage of apple cider vinegar depends on certain factors, including age and health. Make sure that you consult your health care provider prior to the use of apple cider vinegar. Likewise, you should follow the directions indicated on the label or packaging of the product.

The Types of Apple Cider Vinegar

The natural tonic comes in two kinds: filtered and unfiltered.

The filtered variety consists of water and apple cider or juice. Its mother as well as any other sediments have been removed during the filtering process; thus, making it clear and amber-colored. Pasteurizing it further clarifies and refines it.

Unfiltered apple cider vinegar, on the other hand, consists of water and apple cider or juice. However, it still contains the mother and it is not likely to have been pasteurized. It appears to be cloudy and may also have small amounts of sediments.

Basically, the presence of the mother is the only difference between the two. The mother is a murky collection of acetic acid bacteria and cellulose that turns alcohol into vinegar.

If you're going to use apple cider vinegar for cooking purposes, you may go for either of the two types. Both of them have a mild sweetness and an acidic level of five percent. However, if you prefer organic ingredients, you may want to use the unfiltered version since it is most likely to be organically made.

Also, if you want to make your own homemade vinegar, you should go for the unfiltered version since it contains the mother. Plus, it is less processed. So, it is ideal if you prefer less refined foods or are conscious about your health.

Then again, if you are on a budget, you may want to go for the pasteurized and filtered version. It is less expensive, but it can still give you the flavor as well as health benefits you need from apple cider vinegar.

What about taking it in Pill Form?

Aside from being available in its conventional liquid form, apple cider vinegar is also sold in pill or tablet form (most often available at 285 milligrams each).

However, these supplements do not really contain much vinegar. Hence, it is still better to get the liquid variety. In addition, apple cider vinegar pills raise the risk of esophageal burns. There has been an incident in which a woman got an apple cider vinegar tablet stuck in her throat. The ideal (and safest) way to directly consume apple cider vinegar is to dilute it in water and drink it.

Considerations and Precautions

Before you consume anything, see to it that you find out about any possible safety concerns. Apple cider vinegar is generally safe for everyone, except in certain cases. It can even be used for medical purposes. However, it may be harmful when taken in large doses or applied to the skin. In fact, it may cause chemical burns after just a single use.

Consumption of large doses may result in health issues such as weak bones and low potassium levels. It may also cause pain and tenderness in the voice box when taken in the form of tablets, such as in the case of one woman. After thirty minutes of lodging an apple cider vinegar tablet in her throat, she experienced pain and tenderness in her voice box as well as had difficulty swallowing for six months.

In addition, you have to consider if consuming apple cider vinegar may have certain interactions with medications. As much as possible, you should refrain from taking it along with these medications to avoid unpleasant side effects. Consult your doctor if you have any concerns.

For example, it can have a moderate reaction with digoxin. If you take huge amounts of apple cider vinegar, you may have low potassium levels. This, in turn, may boost the side effects of digoxin. Likewise, the natural tonic isn't recommended to be used with insulin since insulin may also reduce the levels of potassium in the body.

Individuals with diabetes should be careful when taking apple cider vinegar as it may also negatively interact with anti-diabetes drugs, such as glimepiride, glyburide, insulin, rosiglitazone, pioglitazone, glipizide, chlorpropamide, and tolbutamide among others.

These medications are typically used to lower blood sugar levels. Hence, taking them with apple cider vinegar may cause your blood sugar to become very low. If you do decide to take it together with these drugs, closely monitor your blood sugar. You may have to change the dose of your anti-diabetes medication (you'll have to talk to your doctor about this).

In addition, you should be careful when taking water pills or diuretic drugs, such as chlorothiazide, furosemide, and hydrochlorothiazide, with apple cider vinegar. Take note that both of them can lower the levels of potassium in the body. Hence, taking them at the same time can cause the mineral's levels to be too low.

CHAPTER 2:
Detoxing and Cleansing Your Body

Consuming apple cider vinegar on a regular basis can help with weight loss, balance the pH level of the body, reduce appetite, and improve digestion. It can also positively affect cholesterol and blood sugar levels, as well as improve the immune system, produce enzymes, heal skin conditions, help flush out toxins, and provide probiotics to the gut.

Because of these great benefits, more and more people are starting to include apple cider vinegar in their daily routine and lifestyle. With regular exercise and a balanced diet, the consumption of this natural health tonic can significantly improve your health and wellness.

Your body has amazing detox systems that encourage waste product removal. Your liver and kidneys, for instance, filter such waste to ensure that your body functions at its best. Unfortunately, there are certain foods that tend to interfere with the natural detoxification process. This is why you have to evaluate your diet and modify it if necessary—such as through the addition of apple cider vinegar.

Detoxing Your Body: A Quick Overview

Whether you want to lose weight or have more energy, detoxing your body will give you plenty of benefits.

For starters, it can help you start a better diet. Even though you do not eat healthily a hundred percent of the time, you can still avoid diseases when you add apple cider vinegar to your diet. After all, there are times when you just have to have a sweet treat or grab a slice of pizza for a quick lunch.

Detox can also kick-start weight loss. If you feel like you've already done everything to lose weight and yet you still do not see positive results, you can try detoxing with apple cider vinegar. It can help you lose the first few pounds, making you feel motivated to continue your weight loss journey.

If energy is your main concern though, you'll be glad to know that detoxing can give you a boost. Some people think that eating will make them more energetic. While it is true that consuming food provides your body the energy it needs to function properly, consuming the wrong types of food will only make it lethargic.

For example, junk foods that contain refined sugars and have low nutritional value can give you a quick energy boost. In the long run, however, these will cause your blood sugar level to spike and crash. This, in turn, will cause you to become more irritable, fatigued, and unable to concentrate. It will also make you crave for unhealthy foods.

By detoxing, you can eliminate those unhealthy choices and get a natural energy boost from the right eats.

What about Apple Cider Detox? Is It Any Better?

Today, there are so many different detox diet plans available. Each and every one of them has its own pros and cons. It can be pretty difficult to find out which is the most ideal as well as what its negative side effects are. Nevertheless, the apple cider vinegar detox is fuss-free and simple.

More importantly though, this approach to detoxification and cleansing is actually supported by science. Here are a few interesting findings regarding the natural tonic's effects and potency:

Effects on Weight Loss

In 2007, researchers have found that consuming apple cider vinegar results in weight loss.

They worked with individuals who had type-1 diabetes. Ten of these participants were served with pudding and a cup of water that contained two tablespoons of apple cider vinegar.

After the study, the participants who consumed apple cider vinegar had slower rates of gastric emptying. Thus, they felt fuller for longer periods of time, causing them to reduce their food intake and helping them achieve weight loss.

Effects on Cholesterol

In 2009, Japanese researchers discovered that consuming vinegar caused weight loss in animals. They also learned that this simple practice can affect triglyceride and cholesterol levels. Triglycerides are the fatty acids present in the blood.

In another study, Iranian researchers suggested that apple cider vinegar may also reduce bad cholesterol or LDL, triglycerides, and total cholesterol in individuals with high cholesterol levels.

Effects on Blood Sugar

Consuming apple cider vinegar with food may also help regulate blood sugar levels. When you eat foods that are rich in carbohydrates, your blood sugar levels may go up. However, drinking less than an ounce of apple cider vinegar after eating a meal that's rich in carbohydrates can help stabilize your blood glucose levels.

In a study that involved individuals with type-2 diabetes, it was found that taking apple cider vinegar with midnight snacks can slow down the rate at which carbohydrate is converted into sugar. This was due to the acetic acid found in apple cider vinegar.

In the study, the participants consumed two tablespoons of apple cider vinegar along with cheese snacks. Upon waking up in the morning, they were found to have had lower blood sugar levels.

What about the Possible Side Effects?

Just like everything else, apple cider vinegar may be harmful if used in excessive amounts. See to it that you educate yourself about the potential risks of apple cider vinegar before you consume it.

For instance, too much of it can erode the tooth enamel. In order to prevent this from happening, you have to limit your consumption and use a straw when drinking it. You should also take it with food or mix it with water. Do not forget to rinse your mouth after consuming it.

Aside from that, apple cider vinegar may interact with certain supplements and medications, such as insulin and diuretics. If you are using any prescription medication, see to it that you consult your doctor before taking apple cider vinegar.

Keep in mind that apple cider vinegar is highly acidic. It may irritate your stomach and throat. Thus, you should refrain from taking it on an empty stomach. If you ever experience throat irritation, you should immediately drink a glass of water.

How to Detox Using Apple Cider Vinegar

Ideally, you should use raw and unfiltered apple cider vinegar with the mother. It contains minerals, probiotics, and enzymes that are good for your health.

You need one to two tablespoons of apple cider vinegar, eight ounces of water, and an optional one to two tablespoons of sweetener. You may use honey, stevia, or maple syrup. You can put apple cider vinegar in your salad dressing and marinades for vegetables and meats. Likewise, you can spray it onto popcorn, mix it with green juices, and stir it into stews and soups.

Depending on your health and fitness goal, you may consume apple cider vinegar for a few days or a month. You may also repeat the detox several times per year. What's important, however, is that you try it for at least three days—that's enough time for you to see its amazing results.

Proper Dietary Choices: Foods to Eat and Avoid

As much as possible, you should eat a lot of vegetables and fruits. Ideally, you should have five to eight portions per day. You also need to load up on nuts, whole grains, seeds, and healthy fats such as olive oil. Eat moderate amounts of eggs and lean meats. And yes, drinking herbal teas is recommended.

On the other hand, you should steer clear of fatty meats, sugars, and refined grain products such as white rice, pasta, and white bread. You have to avoid high-fat dairy products such as butter and cream. Likewise, stay away from processed foods and fried foods, as well as caffeinated drinks. These unhealthy food choices contribute to fatigue, digestive problems, sluggishness, and weight gain.

10 Amazing Drink Recipes for a Quick Detox

Cleanse drinks or detox drinks help improve bodily function by getting rid of toxins and free radicals. They also aid in weight loss. However, it is not advisable to consume these beverages alone for more than a week. Make sure that you also consult your doctor before you begin.

Keep in mind that these detox drinks are only supplementary to a healthy diet. If you want to be fitter and healthier, you should eat nutritious foods and exercise on a regular basis. Nonetheless, it is ideal to consume these beverages in the morning along with your breakfast. Here are some recipes you can try:

Cucumber Mint Detoxing Drink

Mint is a natural cure for stomachaches. It also speeds up digestion by improving the flow of bile in the stomach. When combined with cucumber, it becomes the perfect drink for a warm sunny day.

Ingredients:
- 9 mint leaves
- 1 cucumber
- 2 tablespoons apple cider vinegar
- Black rock salt
- Water
- Ice cubes

Instructions:
1. Peel and slice the cucumber into several pieces. Place them in a blender.
2. Add the mint leaves and water. Blend the ingredients.
3. Strain the mixture and discard the pulp.
4. Add some black rock salt and apple cider vinegar. Dilute with water if necessary.
5. Pour the mixture in a glass and add some ice cubes.

Orange Carrot Ginger Detoxing Drink

Oranges are rich in vitamin C and antioxidants. Carrots are rich in fiber and beta-carotene. Gingers have anti-inflammatory properties that make them ideal for digestion problems, bloating, and stomach cramps.

Ingredients:

- 2 oranges
- 1 carrot
- ½ lemon
- 1 tablespoon apple cider vinegar
- ½ inch ginger
- ½ inch raw turmeric

Instructions:

1. Crush the ginger and turmeric.
2. Juice the carrot and orange separately.
3. Pour the juices in your blender.
4. Add the crushed ginger, turmeric, and apple cider vinegar.
5. Blend the ingredients for thirty seconds. Squeeze half a lemon over it.
6. Strain the mixture and serve.

Pomegranate Juice

This detoxing drink mainly consists of beetroot and pomegranate. It also contains aloe vera, which further increases its effectiveness in improving the immune system.

Ingredients:

- 2 cups pomegranate juice
- 1 tablespoon apple cider vinegar
- ½ cup chopped beetroot
- 1 aloe vera leaf
- ¼ teaspoon black pepper

Instructions:

1. Peel off the aloe vera rind and discard it.
2. Peel off the yellow layer beneath this rind to reveal the clear gel. Scrape off about two tablespoons of this gel. Clean it.
3. Place the pomegranate juice, apple cider vinegar, and beetroot in your blender. Blend the ingredients.
4. Add the aloe vera gel to the mixture. Blend the ingredients once more.
5. Add the black pepper. Serve and enjoy.

Radiant Lemonade

Lemon water detox is highly popular amongst fitness enthusiasts. It is said to be rich in pectin fiber, which keeps you full for longer periods of time. This detoxing drink mainly consists of apples, carrots, radish, and beetroot. It also contains lemon juice for a nice citrus boost.

Ingredients:
- 1 carrot
- 1 apple
- 2 lemons
- 2 slices white radish
- ½ beetroot
- ½ teaspoon lemon zest
- 1 tablespoon apple cider vinegar

Instructions:
1. Chop the carrot and the apple. Slice the beetroot and juice the lemons.
2. Combine all ingredients in your blender.
3. Blend away, adding some water if necessary.
4. Sieve the mixture. Serve and enjoy.

Honey Lemon Ginger Tea

Tea has long been renowned for its health benefits. When you add honey, lemon, and ginger to it, it becomes an effective natural remedy for cold and sore throat. It also becomes a delicious and nutritious detoxing drink.

Ingredients:
- 1 teaspoon honey
- 1 teaspoon lemon juice
- 1 teaspoon apple cider vinegar
- 1 teaspoon ginger
- 1 teaspoon tea leaves
- 3 cups water

Instructions:
1. Heat three cups of water in a pan.
2. Chop the ginger and add it to the water before it boils.
3. Add the honey, tea leaves, and lemon juice when the water begins to boil.
4. Mix in the apple cider vinegar then strain the mixture into a cup.

Coconut Water with Mint and Lemon

This delightful detoxing drink will free your liver and intestinal tract from toxins, leaving you fresh and energetic. It only takes fifteen minutes to make.

Ingredients:
- 1 lemon
- 1 coconut
- 1 tablespoon honey
- 1 tablespoon apple cider vinegar
- Mint leaves

Instructions:
1. Open the coconut and pour its juice into a container.
2. Using a spoon, scrape off the coconut meat.
3. Chop the coconut meat finely. Add it to the coconut water.
4. Add the lemon, lemon juice, mint, apple cider vinegar, and honey.
5. Stir all ingredients together. Serve and enjoy.

Ginger Litchi Lemonade

Ginger has anti-inflammatory properties, enabling it to cleanse your organs and improve your health. With this flavorful summer cooler, you get to refresh and nourish your body at the same time.

Ingredients:
- ½ cup lemon juice
- ½ cup ginger
- ½ cup chia seeds
- 1 cup grapes
- 1 glass lychee juice
- 1 tablespoon apple cider vinegar
- Salt
- Mint leaves
- Ice cubes

Instructions:
1. Mince the ginger. Put it in a jar.
2. Add the lychee and lemon juices, then add the apple cider vinegar.
3. Add the salt and ice cubes. Shake everything to mix them well.
4. Pour the beverage into a glass. Add chia seeds and sliced grapes. Stir with a spoon.
5. Garnish it with mint leaves. Serve chilled.

Aam Panna

It's made with mango pulp, cumin, mint leaves, and jeera. It is both energizing and refreshing. This drink is definitely perfect for summer. It will keep you hydrated and cool during hot days.

Ingredients:
- 2 cups water
- 2 tablespoons chopped mint leaves
- 2 teaspoons cumin seeds (roasted and powdered)
- 2 teaspoons black rock salt
- 1 tablespoon apple cider vinegar
- ½ cup sugar
- 500 grams green mangoes

Instructions:
1. In a pot, boil the mangoes until they become soft and their skin changes color.
2. Let the mangoes cool. When they are cool enough, remove their skin. Squeeze out their pulp.
3. Combine all ingredients in a container. Add two cups of water.
4. Get a glass and put some ice cubes in it. Pour the beverage over it.

Fruit Infused Tea

This exquisite tea blend combines berries, orange, mint leaves, ginger, and chamomile. It is detoxifying and rejuvenating.

Ingredients:
- 2 cups boiling water
- 2 chamomile tea bags
- 8 mint leaves
- 1 orange
- 1 tablespoon apple cider vinegar
- 10 grams ginger
- 50 grams blueberries
- 50 grams other berries of your choice

Instructions:
1. Brew the chamomile tea along with the berries, mint leaves, ginger, and orange rind for four minutes.
2. Pour the beverage into a tea cup. Serve hot.

Detox Haldi Tea

This detoxing drink has anti-inflammatory and antioxidative properties. Its primary ingredient, turmeric, is a powerful spice that cleanses the liver and boosts immune function.

Ingredients:
- 2 cups water
- 1 teaspoon honey
- ¼ teaspoon black pepper
- ½ teaspoon chopped ginger
- ½ teaspoon haldi
- 1 tablespoon apple cider vinegar

Instructions:
1. Boil the water in a pot.
2. Add the ingredients and stir.
3. Continue boiling the liquid until it is reduced by half.
4. Pour the haldi tea into a cup. Mix in the apple cider vinegar. Serve.

CHAPTER 3:
Using Nature's Tonic for Body Care

As made clear so far, apple cider vinegar has plenty of health benefits to offer. In fact, it can even serve as a natural cure for everything, from infections to diabetes. Plus, it can significantly improve both fitness and lifestyle. Here's something you probably didn't expect though—aside from ingesting apple cider vinegar, you can use it externally to care for the skin.

Yes, the so-called natural tonic has been found to be beneficial for skin problems. It has antimicrobial properties that help soothe irritation and treat skin infections. It can likewise help restore your skin's natural pH, allowing it to keep irritants out and moisture in. Thus, apple cider vinegar should be a great addition to your daily skin care routine.

Putting a Stop to Skin-related Issues

Truth be told, vinegar has always been the go-to solution for a variety of medical dilemmas. For centuries, people from all over the world have used it for medicinal purposes. At present, experts still recommend it for health issues, including skin conditions such as eczema, dandruff, and yeast infections.

Studies continue to support and further prove the notion that apple cider vinegar can be used to treat infections caused by bacteria. The following are some of the conditions that may benefit from the use of this fascinating product:

Bacterial Vaginosis and Yeast Infections

Bacterial vaginosis and yeast infections are both caused by an overgrowth of microbes in the vagina. Such infections occur when bad bacteria overrun their beneficial counterparts.

In 2018, researchers conducted a study involving the body's external regions. They found that apple cider vinegar inhibits the growth of Candida (a yeast) and certain types of bacteria. They also found that apple cider vinegar increases its power against yeast when combined with water by a ratio of 1:1.

Likewise, they discovered that apple cider vinegar maintains its power against E.coli and Staphylococcus when diluted by 1:50 and 1:25 ratios. Hence, it can be said that adding it to a partially filled bathtub can help fight against infections.

Body Odor

Apple cider vinegar can kill certain types of bacteria outside the body. It's an effective alternative to deodorants. Adding it in your bath can help prevent body odor.

Eczema

The skin has a natural barrier that is quite acidic. When it becomes less acidic, moisture is able to escape from the skin, causing it to become dry. This barrier also protects the skin against irritants.

According to researchers, individuals with eczema have a higher skin pH. This means that the protective barrier of their skin is not acidic enough. Since apple cider vinegar is a mild acid, applying it topically can help restore the skin's protective barrier.

Dandruff

There are several causes of dandruff, including Malassezia, a yeast-like fungus. Since apple cider vinegar has antifungal properties, it may kill off this fungus. If things are getting flaky, you can dip your scalp in an apple cider vinegar bath to get relief.

Dry Skin

Researchers have found that the more acidic your skin is, the healthier it becomes. The protective layer of your skin allows it to retain moisture. When you wash your skin with water and soap, it becomes less acidic.

So, if you have dry skin, you should occasionally soak your body in an apple cider vinegar bath to retain its natural acidity and prevent damage and further dryness.

Athlete's Foot

Fungal infection causes athlete's foot. Vinegar has antifungal properties. In fact, it is a well-known natural remedy for nail fungus. Hence, using apple cider vinegar on your foot can help treat this condition.

Varicose Veins

Varicose veins may cause leg fatigue, leg cramps, itching, and pain. Applying apple cider vinegar topically may reduce the symptoms associated with these varicose veins.

Warts and Pimples

Apple cider vinegar may be directly applied to pimples to help eliminate pore-clogging bacteria. It may likewise be applied to warts to burn them away. Moreover, it can be added to baths to help prevent warts and pimples from developing.

Apple Cider Vinegar: A Versatile Solution

Apple cider vinegar can be made into a bath, a foot bath, and a remedy for razor burn. If you have some skin-related concerns, such as those just mentioned, you can help your body by taking an apple cider vinegar bath.

You need to mix ¼ cup of sea salt, ¼ cup of baking soda, and ¼ cup of Epsom salt. Fill up your bathtub with warm water and add 1/3 cup of apple cider vinegar. Pour in the dry mixture of salts and baking soda. You can also add some essential oils if you want.

A solution composed only of water and apple cider vinegar should be still be fine, especially if don't have the other ingredients available. Just follow these steps to make a simple apple cider vinegar bath:

1. Fill up your bathtub with warm water (it has to be warm, not hot).

2. Pour two cups of raw apple cider vinegar into the water.

3. Stir the mixture with your hand.

Regardless of which formula you choose to follow, once you're done preparing it you can get into the bathtub and soak yourself for fifteen to twenty minutes. Afterwards, you should take a shower to rinse.

Of course, you could try other ratios in preparing your rejuvenating bath, though this is something that should be done carefully and gradually. So, begin with the most common recommendations. Also, keep in mind that making your bath too acidic won't help your skin at all.

By the way, if you live in a place where the weather is warm, chances are you have athlete's foot or stinky feet. Don't worry because you can treat such problems using apple cider vinegar. To prepare this remedy, simply mix 4 cups of water and 1 cup of apple cider vinegar. You can use your bathtub or even a pot, as long as your feet can fit inside. When the mixture is ready, you can soak your feet for fifteen minutes. Afterwards, you can rinse and dry.

You can also use apple cider vinegar to treat razor burns. Simply dip a cotton ball into a small amount of apple cider vinegar and then directly apply it on the affected area. If you have sensitive skin, you can apply some honey on the region and let it set before you apply apple cider vinegar.

CHAPTER 4:
Other Uses of Apple Cider Vinegar

Studies have shown that this natural tonic has plenty of uses and offers loads of benefits. It can facilitate weight loss, lower blood sugar levels, improve symptoms of diabetes, reduce cholesterol, and support skin health, among others. It is also commonly used for cooking and household purposes.

To give you a better idea of just how versatile it really is, here are some of its other fascinating applications:

In the Kitchen

For pickling vegetables

Fermented foods are great. They are ideal to be served in picnics and parties. You can add apple cider vinegar to quick pickles as well as use it for flavor at the end of the fermentation process.

For marinades and salad dressings

You can use it to add flavor to your marinades and salad dressings.

To make buttermilk

If you're vegan, you probably have a hard time shopping for groceries. Worry no more because apple cider vinegar is an excellent ingredient for nearly everything in your diet.

If you want buttermilk, however, you can make your own by mixing one teaspoon of apple cider vinegar with a plant-based milk. Let the mixture sit for five minutes and enjoy your gluten-free buttermilk.

For making poached eggs

If you like poached eggs but you find them difficult to prepare, using apple cider vinegar can make things easier for you. If you add some apple cider vinegar to the water, the egg whites will become firmer faster. This technique also helps in minimizing the mess you make while cooking.

For enhancing your braising liquid

You can add two tablespoons of apple cider vinegar to your braised meats and vegetables to make them tastier.

For better bone broths

If you like broths, you can add one to two tablespoons of apple cider vinegar to your bone broth to make it healthier. This product helps pull minerals and nutrients from the bones into the water.

To boil eggs more easily

If you like boiled eggs, you can use apple cider vinegar to speed up the process as well as ensure that the eggs maintain their shape. This is especially helpful if the eggs crack when they boil. Adding apple cider vinegar to the water will firm up the egg white as soon as possible; thus, preventing it from spilling out of the shell.

For candies and cakes

If you like to cook and bake, you can use apple cider vinegar to improve the texture and flavor of your food. This is especially ideal for vegan treats since they cannot contain eggs. Apple cider vinegar can also make homemade caramels more flavorful.

For rinsing vegetables and fruits

To ensure that you get rid of any traces of pesticides on your vegetables and fruits, you can use apple cider vinegar to wash them. This is so much better than washing them with water alone. In fact, studies have shown that washing food in vinegar effectively removes bacteria such as salmonella and E. coli.

To clean dishes

You can use apple cider vinegar to rinse dirty dishes instead of a regular dish soap. Its antibacterial properties will ensure that your dishes are clean and safe to use. And by the way, you can simply add apple cider vinegar to your dishwasher.

Personal Care

As a tooth whitener

If your teeth are stained, you can restore their whiteness by applying a mixture of baking soda, water, and apple cider vinegar. This works due to the abrasive effect of apple cider vinegar. In fact, some say that using nature's tonic alone, rubbing it directly on one's teeth, provides better results. While that's likely to be true, there's the issue of harming the enamel and ending up with weaker teeth.

To fight against bad breath

Instead of a regular mouthwash, you can use apple cider vinegar to rinse your mouth and freshen your breath. This product contains acetic acid that fights against bacteria. You can rinse or gargle with one tablespoon of apple cider vinegar mixed with warm water.

For cleaning toothbrushes

Aside from keeping your teeth white and your breath fresh, apple cider vinegar can also clean your toothbrush. To make a homemade cleaner, you have to mix two tablespoons of apple cider vinegar with two teaspoons of baking soda and half a cup of water. Submerge the head of your toothbrush into this mixture and leave it there for half an hour before rinsing.

For cleaning dentures

If you have dentures, you can wash them with apple cider vinegar to make sure that they are clean and fresh. This is considered to be less harmful to the skin in the mouth than any other cleaning agents.

As a shampoo

Likewise, you can use apple cider vinegar to wash your hair instead of a regular shampoo. This works just as well as the shampoos you see in grocery stores. It can revitalize your scalp, all while detangling your hair and making it shinier. You can mix two tablespoons of apple cider vinegar with eight ounces of water to rinse your hair.

As a skin toner

Daily exposure to the sun, smoke, and dust takes a toll on your skin. Hence, you should try using apple cider vinegar to rebalance your skin's pH and remove oil. The natural tonic also has antibacterial properties that can help eliminate acne.

To make an apple cider vinegar skin toner, you have to mix two parts of water and one part of apple cider vinegar. Use a cotton pad to apply the mixture on your face. If you have sensitive skin, you should use more water.

As a body scrub

If you are getting tired of expensive, unnatural body scrubs, you'll be glad to know that the all-natural tonic can be made into an excellent substitute. Simply combine two tablespoons of it with a tablespoon of honey and a cup of granulated sugar. Honey is known to fight microbes, provide antioxidants, and improve complexion. Granulated sugar, on the other hand, draws moisture into the skin while also serving as an exfoliant.

As a foot deodorizer

You can mix apple cider vinegar with Epsom salt and water to deodorize your feet. This will kill odor-causing bacteria and eliminate unpleasant foot odor.

To deodorize your underarms

Instead of using a commercial deodorant, you can dilute apple cider vinegar in water and apply the solution onto your underarms. This would keep you feeling fresh and odor-free all day long.

Health Matters

As treatment for Candida overgrowth

Apple cider vinegar has antifungal properties that may also help you treat Candida.

As treatment for toenail and foot fungi

Rather than go to your local drugstore to purchase medication for your toenail and foot fungi, you can try using apple cider vinegar. Simply mix it with water and soak your feet in it for a while. Do this daily until your condition gets better.

To add to your sitz bath

If you are suffering from hemorrhoids, you can experience relief by taking a sitz bath with apple cider vinegar. Simply mix cold or warm water with ¼ cup of apple cider vinegar and add it to your sitz bath.

To soothe sore throat

If you have sore throat, you can turn to apple cider vinegar for relief instead of relying on sore throat medication. Apple cider vinegar has antibacterial properties that make it just as effective as traditional medications for a variety of ailments, including sore throat.

To make this home remedy, you need to dilute the apple cider vinegar in water and then use the mixture to gargle or rinse your throat. Keep in mind that apple cider vinegar is highly acidic. Thus, it is not ideal to be used on its own. It may cause throat burns if not diluted with water.

To help you feel full quickly

If you are trying to lose weight or you want to avoid bloating, you should consume apple cider vinegar. According to researchers, this product is effective in helping people eat fewer calories, reduce belly fat, and lose weight.

As a digestive aid

You can use apple cider vinegar to encourage your stomach to produce acid and aid in the digestive process. You can directly consume one teaspoon of this product or dilute it with water. Take greater amounts if necessary.

As a morning primer

Energize yourself in the morning by drinking eight ounces of water with one to two tablespoons of apple cider vinegar. When you start your day right, you will be more productive, efficient, and happier.

Drinking apple cider vinegar first thing in the morning can prime your kidneys, balance the pH of your body, give you an energy boost, and control microbial balance in your gut.

Home Upkeep

To get rid of unpleasant odors

Since apple cider vinegar has antibacterial properties, it can be used as a deodorizer to keep your home smelling fresh. Mix water and apple cider vinegar to make a deodorizing spray for your home. This makes it an excellent natural alternative to the odor neutralizers sold in stores.

As a home cleaning product

When you mix apple cider vinegar with baking soda, essential oils, and water, you can have a powerful all-purpose cleaner for your home. Unlike the cleaning products you see in the grocery store, this homemade cleaner is non-toxic yet effective.

As a weed repellent

Rather than use a commercial pesticide and herbicide laced with chemicals, you should use a mixture of water and apple cider vinegar to get rid of weeds in your garden. If this weed killer solution isn't enough to get things done, you should consider the following options:

• *Using pure apple cider vinegar*
  › As you can surely imagine, the higher acidity of vinegar alone (compared to the vinegar-water solution) is more detrimental to weed.

• *Combining apple cider vinegar with soap*
  › This requires you to add an ounce of soap (dishwashing detergent) for every gallon of vinegar. Although really potent at killing weed, this is also harmful to insect life and other plants. So, be very careful when applying this in your garden.

• *Adding both detergent and salt*
  › There are cases in which even the vinegar-and-soap solution fails to yield results. This is where you may want to add salt into the mix. Salt is even more harmful to plants since it ruins water balance at a cellular level, dehydrating even the toughest of weed. To prepare this improved solution, just mix together a cup of salt, a gallon of vinegar, and a tablespoon of soap.

To eliminate pet fleas

Do not let your pet suffer from fleas. However, you should not expose it to harmful chemicals either. Instead of using a commercial product, you can use a mixture of water and apple cider vinegar to get rid of those pesky parasites. Combine one part water and one part apple cider vinegar, and then apply the resulting concoction on the fur of your pet.

A good rule of thumb is to test a small part first to see if your pet has a reaction towards the mixture. If your pet does not experience discomfort or develop allergies, you can use the mixture throughout its body.

To keep fruit flies away

You can mix apple cider vinegar with water and dish soap in a bowl. Then, you should leave the mixture in the kitchen to keep the fruit flies away.

To wash away cat urine

If you have cats at home, you have probably had the trouble of washing clothes with your pets' urine. While it's just a territorial thing to your feline friends, there's no denying that the odor is far from pleasant. With apple cider vinegar, you won't have to rely on chemical cleansers and detergents to make your clothes smell fresh again.

The entire process is actually quite simple. Dilute a cup of apple cider vinegar in three cups of water. Soak your clothes in this concoction for several minutes. Afterwards, wash your clothes with cold water (there's no need to use soap). Finally, dry your clothes as you would normally. If there is still a lingering smell, you may have to repeat the process a few more times.

CHAPTER 5:
Apple Cider Vinegar and Diet Plans

When apple cider is fermented by bacteria and yeast, apple cider vinegar is produced. This liquid has turned the sugars into alcohol and then into acetic acid. Apple cider vinegar is typically labelled raw, filtered, and organic.

Apple cider vinegar is rich in enzymes and probiotics. It contains amino acids, live enzymes, malic acid, acetic acid, and pectin among others. One serving of this tonic has zero fat, minimal salt and sugars, and only three calories. It also contains manganese, iron, selenium, sodium, phosphorus, magnesium, potassium, and calcium.

With this being said, you can conclude that apple cider vinegar is truly good for your health. So, where can you fit it in your everyday diet? It is actually suitable for individuals on certain diets, such as keto, paleo, autoimmune protocol (AIP), and candida, since it fits a lot of dietary restrictions.

Apple Cider Vinegar and the Keto Diet

The ketogenic diet, also commonly referred to as the keto diet, is a meal plan that puts emphasis on keeping carbs to a minimum. It's typically followed by people who aim to lose weight fast.

In essence, the keto diet alters the fuel supply of the body. When you reduce your consumption of carbohydrates, you encourage your body to switch from its usual source of fuel to fat. The keto diet makes your body burn fat for energy through the metabolic process known as ketosis.

The keto diet has three variations: standard, cyclical, and targeted.

The standard keto diet focuses on high fat, moderate protein, and very low carbohydrate intake. The cyclical keto diet follows the principles of the standard keto diet, except that it incorporates carb loading as well. Carb loading occurs when you consume high carbohydrate foods on certain days. The targeted keto diet is about eating foods rich in carbohydrates an hour before exercising. This way, the carbohydrates are used for fuel during the workout.

While on the keto diet, you're only allowed to eat certain types of food. So, you have to train yourself to get used to this new lifestyle. As much as possible, you should plan your meals and make a list of your groceries. Keep in mind that you need get foods that are low in carbs, high in fat, and moderate in protein.

You can eat meats, poultry, seafood, fish, dairy, eggs, seeds, nuts, natural fats, healthy oils, and low-carb vegetables and fruits. Opt for grass-fed meats as much as possible. Refrain from eating nuts that are coated with sugar.

Conversely, you should avoid foods and beverages that contain a lot of carbohydrates and sugars, such as grains, processed foods, starchy vegetables, dried fruits, soda, and alcohol. Avoid anything that is not natural. You should also avoid low-fat foods since you have to aim for high fat intake with the keto diet.

See to it that you include apple cider vinegar in your diet. Following the keto diet can help you regulate your blood sugar levels. As you know, apple cider vinegar has properties that can help you achieve this fitness goal too.

During the times when you cycle out of ketosis and consume a high carb meal, you become at risk of inflammation. This happens because of the insulin increase and the temporary burning of sugar for fuel.

Hence, you need apple cider vinegar to help balance your blood sugar response. According to studies, apple cider vinegar can reduce the glycemic index of a meal that is rich in carbohydrates. Still, you should opt for low glycemic carbohydrate sources instead of white breads.

Ketosis is also the physiological state of oxidizing or burning fat for energy. When you improve the way your body oxidizes fat, you support the state of ketosis. Studies have shown that apple cider vinegar can moderately boost the effects of fat oxidation in your body. This is why some people are able to lose excess body fat when they include apple cider vinegar in their diets.

Take note that the keto diet is generally higher in fat than the diets that most individuals are used to. So, if you have always eaten meats and carbohydrates all your life, your body may need additional support when it breaks down your meals.

A lot of people do not produce enough stomach acid, and that's why they experience problems with digestion. If you are one of these people, consuming apple cider vinegar before meals may prove to be beneficial since it can improve gallbladder function and promote the production of stomach acid.

Furthermore, apple cider vinegar can help you curb carb and sugar cravings. As you know, foods that are high in sugars and carbohydrates can negatively affect your health. When you first start the keto diet, you may experience keto flu symptoms. This happens because your body adapts to burning fat. You may have a blood sugar imbalance and start to crave for foods that are packed with carbs.

Apple Cider Vinegar and the Paleo Diet

The primary principle behind the paleo diet is to only consume what people during the Paleolithic era consumed. This means that the diet is limited to vegetables, fruits, and meats. Grains, processed foods, and anything that is sold in fast food chains are not allowed.

Nevertheless, even though apple cider vinegar is not technically paleo, it still goes well with the paleo diet. It is acceptable because it does not contain sugars or gluten. Moreover, as you know, apple cider vinegar promotes weight loss. So, if you are following the paleo diet to lose weight, you should include this product.

Apple cider vinegar can lower your body mass index, body weight, serum triglycerides, and weight circumference. Obese individuals who consumed beverages that contained one to two tablespoons of vinegar per day were able to lose two to four pounds after just twelve weeks.

What's more, apple cider vinegar makes an excellent salad dressing. If you are worried about your meals tasting bland, you should use apple cider vinegar to make them more savory. This product goes well with leafy vegetables and fruits. It's also great with other dressings, such as extra virgin olive oil, lime juice, lemon juice, avocado oil, and rice vinegar. For an even more flavorful meal, you can add garlic, ginger, basil, dill, oregano, mint, mustard, and black pepper.

Apple Cider Vinegar and the Autoimmune Protocol (AIP) Diet

The autoimmune protocol diet mainly concentrates on reducing gut inflammation and healing the immune system. The National Institutes of Health states that more than twenty-three million individuals in the United States suffer from autoimmune disorders every year.

Autoimmunity is actually among the leading causes of deaths in women under sixty-five years of age. Autoimmune disorders generally include conditions that result from the attack of the immune system towards its organs. Thyroiditis, for instance, is an attack to the thyroid gland. Lupus is an attack to the kidneys. Crohn's disease is an attack to the gastrointestinal system, and multiple sclerosis is an attack to the nervous system.

If you have any of these disorders, you can use food medicine to reduce your symptoms, heal gut dysfunction, and decrease inflammation. The autoimmune protocol diet involves nutrient-dense food to help the body cool down its immune system. It eliminates allergenic and inflammatory dietary options.

When you suffer from an autoimmune disease, your digestive tract is not at its best. Thus, the byproducts of the foods you eat leak through the gut barrier into the bloodstream. This causes your immune system to have a reaction.

In order to improve your condition, you should consume meats, vegetables, fruits, coconut milk, fermented foods, and healthy fats. Avoid grains, beans, dairy, eggs, nuts, seeds, fermented soy products, sugars, sugar substitutes, food additives, and alcohol. You should also make it a habit to drink warm water with apple cider vinegar every morning.

Apple Cider Vinegar and the Candida Diet

The candida diet is an anti-inflammatory diet meant to rebalance gut flora and reduce sugar intake. Its main purpose is to reduce Candida overgrowth in the digestive system. While on this diet, you can consume apple cider vinegar and fermented food since they contain healthy bacteria that inhibit the growth of Candida.

Refrain from consuming anything with refined sugars. Do not buy white and brown sugars as well as maple, rice, and corn syrups. Avoid honey and even molasses. Read the labels of food products carefully. Do not get anything with sucrose, maltose, fructose, glucose, polysaccharides, monosaccharides, galactose, sorbitol, lactose, mannitol, and glycogen.

Since fruits contain natural sugars, you should avoid them too. Likewise, you have to refrain from drinking fruit juices. You are also not allowed to consume anything with yeast and gluten, such as baked goods and pasta.

Mushrooms, peanuts, pistachios, peanut butter, alcohol, coffee, root beer, black tea, cheeses, pickled meats, and processed goods must also be eliminated from your grocery list. All kinds of vinegars, except apple cider vinegar, are also not allowed.

You can have an apple cider vinegar cleanse to get rid of the excess yeast in your system and restore the balance in your body. Make sure that your apple cider vinegar contains the mother. Use it two times per day for two weeks to improve your condition.

An Important Reminder

In case you experience any unpleasant symptoms, you should discontinue the diet (whichever you end up choosing) and go see your doctor. Seek advice from your nutritionist or dietitian as well. You might be allergic to certain ingredients or the diet is simply not right for you.

CHAPTER 6:
Quick Review of What We've Learned

As you have learned throughout this book, apple cider vinegar is a positive addition to your diet and lifestyle. It can help you with weight loss and in staying within your ideal weight. In fact, it is used and recommended by many diet gurus and fitness experts. It is even included in many fad diets due to its ability to make the body shed pounds quickly.

Researchers have found that the acetic acid present in apple cider vinegar helps the body suppress fat buildup. In a certain study, the participants took fifteen to thirty milliliters of vinegar diluted in water daily. They were able to achieve a significant reduction in total abdominal fat and waist size.

Apple cider vinegar also contains good bacteria that promote healthy gut flora growth. Its high acetic content balances the body's pH level. When apple cider vinegar goes through the fermentation process, it retains the mother, which is responsible for its cloudy appearance and health benefits. It's the one that helps break down food in the digestive tract by stimulating gut enzymes.

Apple cider vinegar has antifungal, antimicrobial, and antibacterial properties. It helps prevent food poisoning caused by the E. coli bacteria. Likewise, it is an effective treatment for thrush and Candida infections. When this fungus overgrows, it can cause digestive tract issues, as well as gas, nausea, diarrhea, and bloating.

Furthermore, apple cider vinegar is beneficial for diabetes. In today's modern world, diabetes is one of the most prevalent health problems. Each year, more and more people are diagnosed with this disease. Increased blood sugar levels or hyperglycemia is a typical symptom of diabetes. It can lead to more severe health problems.

Fortunately, researchers have found that apple cider vinegar's acetic acid content has an anti-glycemic effect. That's why the all-natural tonic is recommended to people with type 1 or type 2 diabetes.

In one study, the participants were given bread with vinegar. They were able to reduce their blood sugar levels by thirty-one percent. Thus, the researchers concluded that even a minimal amount of vinegar, such as the ones used in salad dressings, can significantly affect the body's glycemic response.

In other studies of people with type 2 diabetes, it was found that consuming vinegar has a positive effect on glycemic levels. The participants digested the vinegar in the evening and produced favorable results the next morning. They were able to achieve a six percent reduction.

Moreover, apple cider vinegar can help with insulin sensitivity. Consuming vinegar can improve the fluctuation of insulin in individuals with insulin resistance or type 2 diabetes.

Of course, apple cider vinegar is also beneficial to the skin. Its antifungal and antibacterial properties can cleanse the epidermis. It's helpful for cleaning wounds and reducing acne as well.

A lot of people use apple cider vinegar as a substitute for commercial antibiotic cream. Many dangerous bacterial strains have grown resistant against antibiotic creams. So, using these products may no longer yield the results that you want. Also, the organic acids in apple cider vinegar may be more effective in fighting against bacteria that cause infections.

When it comes to choosing between organic and non-organic apple cider vinegar, it is better to go for organic. Organic products are generally healthier and safer since they are non-GMO and pesticide-free.

They have also not been processed, so they retain their natural state. Organic apple cider vinegar contains the mother, which is a natural aggregate of bacterium that gives it its cloudy appearance. Non-organic apple cider vinegar, on the other hand, has been pasteurized and stripped of healthy enzymes.

According to one study, organic apple cider vinegar contains ninety-six bacteria while non-organic apple cider vinegar only has seventy-two bacteria. And by the way, the fermentation process significantly affects the aroma of the vinegars.

With all of these being said, you can conclude that apple cider vinegar is indeed a good product. It is safe, effective, and may be used on a regular basis. However, just like everything else in life, it has to be used in moderation to prevent unpleasant consequences. See to it that you use apple cider vinegar along with a balanced diet to achieve the best results.

Conclusion

I hope this book was able to help you to learn everything you want to know about apple cider vinegar. I hope that the topics were organized and detailed enough to provide you with the necessary knowledge as well as skills on how to use it properly.

Likewise, I hope that the recipes I provided were easy enough to follow. These beverages are indeed delicious, refreshing, detoxifying, and nutritious. They're perfect for summer or whenever you feel like having a tasty apple cider based-drink.

Then again, you have to be extra careful if you have pre-existing medical conditions. You may not be allowed by your doctor to take apple cider vinegar if you have certain health issues. Similarly, you may not be permitted to use it if you are pregnant or breastfeeding your child.

Nevertheless, the all-natural tonic is generally safe and ideal for almost everyone else. So, if you receive a go signal from your doctor, this book will surely be helpful.

If you want to significantly improve your health, wellness, and life in general, you should make changes as soon as possible. You can begin by rereading this book and truly understand the topics covered in every chapter. More importantly, see to it that you actually apply the lessons that you learn into your life.

The next step is to put the theories you have learned into practice. Now is the right time to take the steps necessary to improve your life.

I wish you the best of luck!

Made in the USA
Middletown, DE
21 August 2019